Hysterect Vaginal R and Surgery for Stress Incontinence

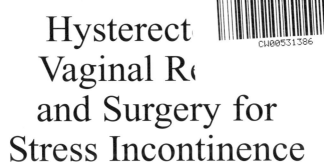

SIXTH EDITION

Sally Haslett
RGN, RM, HvCert

Molly Jennings
MCSP

Hilary Walsgrove
RGN, BSc(Hons), MA

Wendy Weatheritt
MCSP, HPC

BEACONSFIELD PUBLISHERS LTD
Beaconsfield, Bucks, UK

First published 1984
Sixth Edition 2010
Reprinted 2011, 2012, 2013, 2014, 2015, 2016

British Library Cataloguing in Publication Data
A catalogue record for this book is available from the British Library.

ISBN 978–0–906584–62–0

Medical artwork: Barbara Hyams; Oxford Designers & Illustrators
Photography: Mike Messer
Photographic model: Judy Difiore
Phototypeset by Gem Graphics, Trenance, Mawgan Porth, Cornwall in 10¾ on 12¼ Times.
Printed in Great Britain at Halstan & Co. Ltd, Amersham, Bucks.

From the Foreword to the First Edition

Not all doctors are good communicators and many patients in clinics are poor listeners. This is particularly true when they are nervous or worried and faced with the prospect of surgery. At least, many fail to ask all of the questions that may concern them later. When the operation appears to carry the threat of sexual function, the worries can be particularly hard to put into words.

Some years ago in the gynaecological department of St Thomas' Hospital, we attempted to meet this problem by asking two women staff members, who themselves had undergone major gynaecological surgery, to try to explore and relieve the anxieties of women about to have a hysterectomy, or repair surgery for prolapse. The experience was an unqualified success and has contributed greatly to post-operative wellbeing – particularly the long-term mental and physical wellbeing that hospital doctors often ignore.

From this experience Sally Haslett and Molly Jennings have produced this booklet and I recommend that every woman who faces such surgery should now read it. I have no doubt that it will lessen her anxieties and speed her recovery.

R. W. Taylor MD, FRCOG
Professor Emeritus, Department of Obstetrics and Gynaecology
St Thomas' Hospital, London

ACKNOWLEDGEMENTS

We would like to acknowledge with many thanks our indebtedness to the following for their help and support.

The medical staff and senior members of the nursing and physiotherapy staff at St Thomas' Hospital, London for their advice and co-operation in the original development of this booklet.

The following persons, each of whom made time to read a late draft of this Sixth Edition and give us their critical comments, which we were very pleased to be able to take into account when preparing the final version for press: Mr Timothy Hillard, Mrs Heather Betreen, Mrs Diane Kheir and Mrs Pauline Walsh.

S.H., M.J., H.W., W.W.

Contents

INTRODUCTION

When women are advised to have a hysterectomy, a vaginal repair for prolapse, or surgery for stress incontinence they are often reluctant to ask questions about their diagnosis, the surgery to be performed and the convalescent period. This may be due to a lack of understanding of the anatomy of their reproductive organs, but may also be due to embarrassment over the intimate and private nature of their problem. They may simply not know what questions to ask, or feel that what they would like to ask is too basic. It is often easier to obtain this information by having a book to read.

Understanding your reproductive system

First of all, it is important that you should fully understand your anatomy and the terminology used in relation to specific organs (Figures 1, 2 and 3, overleaf). The reproductive organs are contained within the bony pelvis – that is, the ring of bones formed by the two large hip bones, the base of the spine (sacrum) and tail bone (coccyx) at the back and the pubic bones at the front, under the pubic hair. The top rim of the pelvis can be felt about 5 cm (2 inches) below the waist on either side. The reproductive organs are:

The ovaries

The ovaries are situated deep in the pelvis on either side of the womb and contain the eggs for reproduction. In women of child-bearing age, one egg is usually released each month and enters the fallopian tube, where it may become fertilised and pass to the womb.

The fallopian tubes (salpinges)

These open into the womb, one on each side. They are partially lined with little hairs (or cilia) with the ability to help the egg travel along them and enter the womb.

The womb (uterus)

The womb is about the size and shape of a small pear (5–8 cm or 2–3 inches long), wide at the top and narrow below, and lies just behind the pubic bone. It is made up of layers of muscle and is lined with special tissue called endometrium, which has a large blood supply.

1

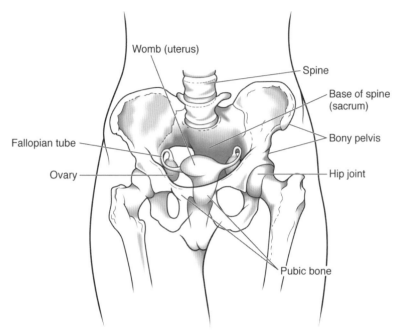

Figure 1 *Front view of female pelvis showing position of womb (uterus) in the body.*

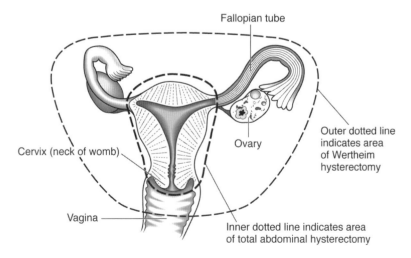

Figure 2 *Front view of womb (uterus).*

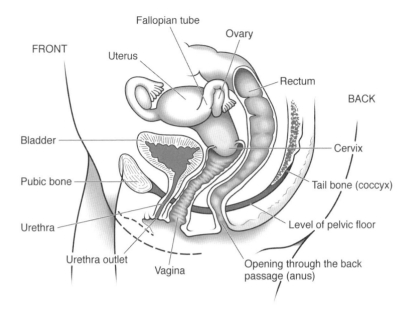

Figure 3   *Side view of female pelvic area, showing pelvic organs and pelvic floor muscles.*

Ligaments which act like ropes hold the womb in position within the pelvis. The function of the womb is to expand to nourish and hold a developing baby. Each month, during a woman's reproductive life, the lining of the womb prepares to receive a fertilised egg for it to implant and grow. If this does not happen, the lining is shed by the normal blood loss of the monthly period (menstruation).

The pelvic floor
The pelvic floor is a 'sling' of muscles and ligaments which support the pelvic organs, including the womb, bladder, urinary canal (urethra) and rectum.

The cervix
The narrow entrance at the 'neck' or base of the womb is called the cervix. This is a ring of muscle that can relax and open to allow a baby to pass through during childbirth.

3

The vagina

The vagina is sometimes called the birth canal and the cervix dips down into it. The vaginal walls are muscular and very elastic, so stretch easily.

The external genitalia (vulva)

The area between the legs into which the vagina opens is called the genitals or vulva. The lips on either side surround the openings from the urethra/urinary canal at the front and from the vagina just behind. The perineum separates the vulva from the anus (Figure 4).

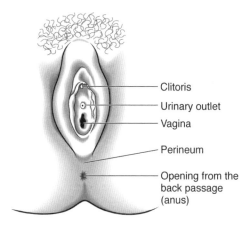

Figure 4   *Female genital area.*

HYSTERECTOMY

Hysterectomy is a surgical operation to remove the womb (uterus). There are a number of different ways that this operation can be carried out and a number of reasons why it might be performed. It is important for a woman to know what sort of hysterectomy she is having and the reasons why it is being carried out. It is unusual for a hysterectomy to be an emergency procedure, which means that there should be some time for a woman and her family and friends to find out exactly what the operation is going to involve in her particular case. It is important to ensure that alternatives to hysterectomy have been explored, in discussion with your doctor, prior to agreement to this operation.

When a hysterectomy is recommended

The doctor should explain fully their decision for this advice and women should be encouraged to ask questions at this stage – even requesting another opinion, if it is felt to be necessary. It is advisable to ask about alternatives to hysterectomy that may be an option for some women but not for others. It may be worth asking about treatments that can postpone the need to have a hysterectomy for short periods of time. This may be an option for a woman who finds it very inconvenient to go ahead with the surgery and the prolonged convalescence required following the operation. However, this is not recommended for women with certain conditions and this needs clarification with your doctor. *It is important to feel fully informed and to understand exactly what the operation means.* You may find it helpful to write down your questions beforehand and possibly take someone with you for support.

A welcome cure

Frequently, symptoms such as heavy bleeding or pain will have been experienced, and a hysterectomy offers a welcome cure and the opportunity of improved health, without affecting a woman's sexuality.

Myths and misconceptions

A hysterectomy is no reason (or excuse!) for gaining or losing weight, neither is it a cause of depression or loss of femininity. Having a hysterectomy should not result in your changing as a person, growing unwanted hair or altering your attitude to sexual relations. These are the type of misconceptions that many women have, prior to going ahead with a hysterectomy. A word of caution! Well-meaning family and friends or even other patients may tell you things that can be alarming and are often inaccurate. Be sensible about this and seek advice from the doctor or nurses.

Coming to terms with hysterectomy

Some women experience difficulty in coming to terms with the prospect of having a hysterectomy. Others find they are affected emotionally after the operation. There may be numerous reasons for this, including social circumstances and cultural and religious beliefs about the female reproductive system and it is important that such issues are addressed. The understanding support of family and friends can be invaluable at this time, but time for discussion with a sympathetic health professional is important and can help to lessen anxiety.

Talking about your hysterectomy

A nurse or other health care professional who is experienced in caring for women who have had a hysterectomy may be available to talk to you. They will be familiar with all sorts of concerns and queries, often of a very embarrassing and sensitive nature. However simple or silly any questions may seem, they can still be discussed with the health care professionals. You should not be afraid or embarrassed to approach the team caring for you, especially if you have any doubts about whether or not you should go ahead with the operation. Hysterectomy is a major surgical operation and you need to be sure you are making the right choices with regard to the treatment of your particular problem. It may be useful to prepare a list of questions or concerns for discussion when you speak to the team caring for you.

Be careful about surfing the internet for information. A list of useful sources of information, additional reading material and recommended websites is given on pages 46–48.

Reasons for needing a hysterectomy

Abnormal vaginal bleeding

Abnormal vaginal bleeding occurs at an inappropriate time or in an excessive amount from that experienced during a woman's normal monthly period. When heavy bleeding occurs this is called *menorrhagia*, which may also include the passing of blood clots. When the bleeding is irregular, does not occur on a regular monthly basis and is possibly prolonged in duration, this is termed *metorrhagia*. Such abnormal bleeding may be due to an obvious cause such as endometriosis or fibroids, although in most cases it is *dysfunctional* – where the cause is uncertain, but may be due to hormone imbalance. In some cases, the problem is due to a bleeding disorder or to a condition such as an underactive thyroid gland. If bleeding is very heavy or prolonged, the woman may become anaemic and complain of tiredness and weakness.

Endometriosis and adenomyosis

Endometriosis refers to a spread of the tissue that lines the womb (endometrium) to areas outside the womb, such as the outer surface of the womb, ovaries, fallopian tubes and supporting ligaments within the pelvis, and it may even be found attached to other internal structures such as the bowel and bladder. Adenomyosis is the term used when this displaced tissue is located within the muscle layer (*myometrium*) of the womb. This tissue attempts to shed blood when the woman is having a period as the tissue is under the same hormonal control as the endometrial tissue within the womb. This can lead to the formation of painful cysts ('chocolate cysts') and scarring may result. A woman may experience heavy and painful periods or other less specific symptoms. It is not known why endometriosis and adenomyosis develop, but neither of them is a cancerous condition.

Fibroids (also known as myomas or leiomyomas)

Fibroids are a very common reason for performing a hysterectomy and are found in approximately a quarter of women over the age of forty. They are almost always benign (not cancerous), although very rarely a malignant (cancerous) fibroid is identified. They consist of growths of fibrous and muscular tissue, which can either be single, or more commonly, multiple. They can vary from the size of a pea to that of a big melon and can make the womb bulky. The symptoms depend on the position and size of the fibroids. They can cause heavy and painful periods and pressure symptoms in the pelvic area, be a contributory factor to infertility, or there may be no symptoms at all. In addition to hysterectomy, there are also several other operations that can be per-formed to remove fibroids (see 'Alternatives to Hysterectomy', overleaf).

Pelvic inflammatory disease (PID)

This is an infective and inflammatory condition that affects the uterus, tubes or ovaries and may involve more than one organ. It is thought that a great many cases of PID are caused by infection or may be as a result of surgery. After an initial episode, which may cause abdominal pain, vaginal discharge, pain on intercourse or abnormal bleeding, the woman is prone to further episodes and the condition can become chronic. Where her quality of life is severely affected, hysterectomy may be the treatment of choice, but there are no guarantees that this will cure her problems.

Uterine prolapse

As a woman ages, the vaginal supports begin to lose their tone and sag downwards. A prolapse may be described as 'something coming down' in the vagina. It may cause a dragging sensation, backache and difficulty in controlling the bladder and sometimes the bowel, or discomfort during intercourse.

A uterine prolapse occurs when the uterus and cervix descend into the vagina. In severe cases this may be visible outside the vagina, when it is called a procidentia. The operation for this is a vaginal hysterectomy. A 'vaginal repair' is the operation performed to correct a 'prolapse' of either the bladder or bowel (see pages 12–15 for further details).

Other benign conditions

Hysterectomy may be the operation of choice for other reasons, such as benign ovarian cysts or polyps and conditions such as severe pre-menstrual syndrome and severe period pain (*dysmenorrhoea*), but other options should be considered first, depending on the severity of the condition (see 'Alternatives to Hysterectomy', below).

Cancer of the endometrium, fallopian tubes, ovaries, cervix

Although relatively rare and an uncommon reason for carrying out a hysterectomy, cancerous (*malignant*) growths can occur within any of these structures and hysterectomy is usually a necessary part of the treatment, in combination with *radiotherapy* (X-ray treatment), *chemotherapy* (drug treatment) or a combination of both of these. A woman may complain of some unusual bleeding or discharge, increased tummy size, pain, or may in fact have no symptoms. For specific advice or more detailed information, refer to the sources given in 'Additional Reading' (page 48).

Emergency procedure

Very rarely, hysterectomy is performed as an emergency procedure, such as if uncontrolled bleeding occurs during childbirth.

Alternatives to hysterectomy – some treatment options

The treatments for the conditions mentioned opposite are not always a viable option for some women but can provide an alternative to hysterectomy, although they may not offer a long-term solution.

Abnormal vaginal bleeding

Hormonal drug treatments are available, in some cases, which may be in the form of tablets, injections or a special coil (IUS – intrauterine system).

A number of minor procedures are available for some women with heavy periods, such as a transcervical resection of endometrium (TCRE) and endometrial ablation, which can be performed using a number of different techniques. You may wish to discuss these different options with your doctor.

Endometriosis and adenomyosis

Anti-inflammatory medications and hormonal treatments may be helpful. Surgical treatment to remove the abnormal endometrial deposits and any cysts or to divide any scar tissue that has developed may be possible, but does not always provide a long-term solution.

Fibroids

Hormonal treatments are available, such as progesterone, which can decrease bleeding, to help shrink the fibroids, although the effects may only be temporary. In certain circumstances, especially if the woman wishes to maintain her fertility, an operation can be carried out to remove fibroids. This operation is called *myomectomy* and is carried out in a similar way to an abdominal hysterectomy but with the womb left intact after the fibroids have been removed. The practical advice on surgery, recovery and after-care given in this booklet also applies to myomectomy.

Uterine artery embolisation. This is a treatment that does not usually require a general anaesthetic and is carried out in a special X-ray room. The treatment blocks the blood vessels supplying the fibroids within the womb and causes them to shrink. Not all fibroids are suitable for this procedure.

Uterine prolapse

A flexible ring (or pessary) may be inserted into the vagina to help support the prolapsed womb and keep it in the correct anatomical position.

The different types of hysterectomy

Total abdominal hysterectomy

This involves removal of the womb (*uterus*) and includes removal of the neck of the womb (*cervix*) (see Figure 2, page 2). This is carried out by making a cut on the abdomen, which is usually a horizontal 'bikini-line' cut along the pubic hair line (Figure 5a). For some patients it may be necessary to make a vertical cut from underneath the belly button down to the pubic hair line (Figure 5b).

Figure 5   *Incision sites: (a) Bikini line; (b) Vertical line.*

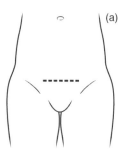 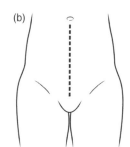

Subtotal hysterectomy

This involves removing the womb but leaving the cervix. As already mentioned, the cervix is the narrow entrance at the base of the womb consisting of a ring of muscle which relaxes and opens when a woman is in labour, to allow the baby to pass through the vagina. For some women the cervix may be involved in orgasm, and if it is removed then they may experience decreased sexual response; however, for many women this is not the case. For women who have had a subtotal hysterectomy, the risk of cervical cancer remains, and they will need to continue to attend for regular smear tests. Leaving the cervix in place may help to prevent prolapse at a later date.

Right or left or bilateral salpingo-oophorectomy (BSO)

Hysterectomy may involve removal of either or both fallopian tubes and either or both ovaries. (*Salpingo* refers to the fallopian tubes and *oophorectomy* refers to the ovaries.) This is likely to be the case if there is a problem with the fallopian tubes or ovaries, or if the woman is approaching the menopause or has already been through the menopause. For women who have not reached menopausal age, it is more usual to leave the ovaries in place, if they are healthy. If the ovaries are suddenly removed from a woman who has not reached the menopause, she is likely to start to experience menopausal symptoms unless the hormones are replaced artificially, i.e. by hormone replacement therapy (HRT) or an alternative therapy (see pages 44–46). This needs to be discussed in detail with the woman prior to a decision being made about removal of the ovaries.

Ovarian conservation

If hysterectomy is carried out before the woman has reached the menopause and the ovaries are left in place, hormones continue to be produced and she is likely to continue to experience the same symptoms that she had during her monthly menstrual cycle, such as breast tenderness, bloating, irritability and so on, but without the monthly bleed. These symptoms, however, are usually less intense than before and will end with the natural menopause (see pages 43–44).

Radical / Wertheim's hysterectomy

When cancer is diagnosed, it may be necessary to perform an extended hysterectomy. This usually involves removing the womb, ovaries and fallopian tubes and may include removal of some adjacent lymph glands, the upper part of the vagina and some of the other surrounding tissue (Figures 2, 3 and 4). In younger women it may be possible to leave the ovaries in place. Everything that is removed will be sent to the pathology laboratory for analysis. Occasionally only a small sample of a suspect area is taken for analysis, which is called a 'biopsy'. As the surgery is more extensive, it is likely to involve a longer hospital stay of approximately seven to ten days. When a cancer has been found, it is sometimes necessary for the woman to have treatment, such as radiotherapy (X-ray treatment) or chemotherapy (drug treatment) or a combination of both, as well as having the hysterectomy. For specific advice or more detailed information, refer to the sources given in 'Additional Reading' (page 48) or ask the doctors and nurses with whom you are in contact.

Vaginal hysterectomy

This is the removal of the womb and the neck of the womb, and is performed through the vagina. This is the operation of choice when there is a 'prolapsed' womb and where repair of the vaginal walls is required at the same time (overleaf). It may also be appropriate to consider a vaginal hysterectomy for other reasons, such as heavy periods, but this method is not normally used if the womb is enlarged, or if the surgeon wishes to look closely at other pelvic or abdominal organs while operating. Occasionally, the ovaries may be removed at the same time by this method. When vaginal surgery is carried out, there is no cut on the abdomen, as the operation is done through the vagina and all the stitches, which are made from a dissolvable material, are on the inside.

Laparoscopic surgery

This means that the surgeon uses a 'keyhole' procedure, by passing a laparoscope (a very fine telescope type of instrument) through a small cut (1–2 cm long) underneath the belly button. There are a number of different ways that a surgeon can perform a hysterectomy using a laparoscopic approach. However, this approach is not always appropriate in particular circumstances. In some cases, laparoscopic hysterectomy has been associated with a shorter hospital stay and recovery than a more traditional abdominal operation. The ovaries may or may not be removed using this approach.

Some risk factors

A hysterectomy is a relatively common operation and is generally safe and successful, but there are risks associated with any type of surgery. Health care staff are very aware of the risks involved and preventative measures are taken to help minimise all potential risk factors. It is important for you to discuss these potential risks and complications with the health care team looking after you.

VAGINAL REPAIR FOR ANTERIOR AND/OR POSTERIOR VAGINAL WALL PROLAPSE

A prolapse occurs when the supporting sling (or ligaments) that holds the womb and other pelvic organs in position is no longer strong enough to do this effectively. The womb may descend or 'drop down' in varying positions, pressing on other pelvic organs such as the bladder or bowel, and resulting in different types of prolapse (Figures 6, 7 and 8). A prolapse may be described as 'something coming down' in the vagina.

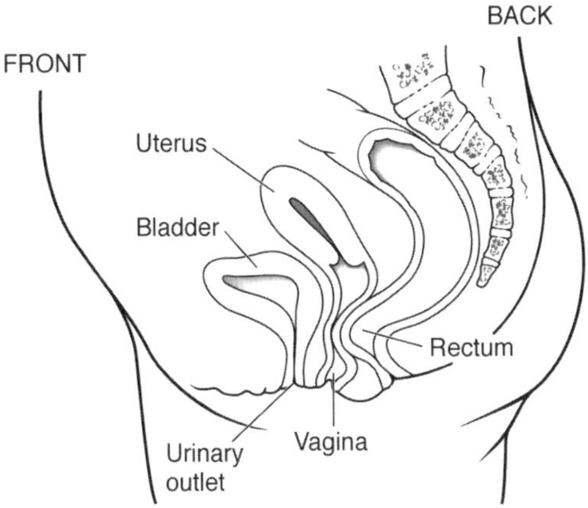

Figure 6   *A rectocele is a bulging of the rectum through the wall of the vagina. An enterocele is a similar problem, possibly involving some of the small bowel, occurring at a higher level than a rectocele. The operation to repair a rectocele is a posterior repair.*

BACK

FRONT

Uterus

Bladder

Rectum

Urinary outlet

Vagina

Figure 7   *A cystocele is a bulging of the bladder through the wall of the vagina. A urethrocele is a bulging of the urethra (urinary passage) through the wall of the vagina. The operation to repair a cystocele is an anterior repair.*

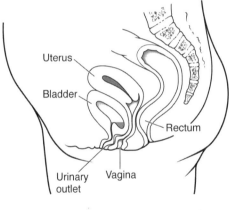

Uterus

Bladder

Rectum

Urinary outlet

Vagina

Figure 8   *A uterine prolapse occurs when the uterus and cervix gradually descend through the vagina. The operation for a uterine prolapse is a vaginal hysterectomy.*

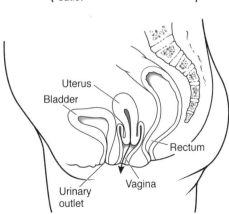

Uterus

Bladder

Rectum

Urinary outlet

Vagina

13

It may cause backache and difficulty in controlling the bladder and sometimes the bowel, or discomfort during sexual intercourse.

Causes of prolapse

The sling (or ligaments), the walls of the vagina and the pelvic floor muscles (Figure 3) have become weakened for various reasons, the most common being pregnancy and childbirth. Other causes may be a chronic cough (as with smokers or people with chest problems), straining when constipated, continuous heavy lifting, or following the menopause when the decrease in production of female hormones effects the elasticity of the tissues.

Vaginal repair

A 'vaginal repair' is an operation performed to correct a 'prolapse'. The surgery to repair a prolapse is often combined with a hysterectomy, in which case the womb is usually removed vaginally and the vaginal walls are strengthened and repaired at the same time, using stitches which dissolve. If the womb is *not* removed, the sling (or ligaments) will be shortened to lift the womb back into place. This will allow the bladder and bowel to return to their correct position. The supporting muscles (pelvic floor muscles) may also need repair due to stretching.

On occasions these muscles and the vaginal walls need repairing at some time *after* a woman has had a hysterectomy.

A repair for prolapse would not ideally be advised until a woman has decided that she does not want any more children. However, 'repair' surgery can be performed without removing the womb. In this case periods, and therefore the possibility of pregnancy, will continue in women who have not yet reached the menopause, and contraception will still be necessary if they are sexually active. If pregnancy does occur, the baby will probably need to be delivered by caesarean section.

Sexual activity

Before the operation, the surgeon needs to know whether or not a woman is sexually active, as this may make a difference to how they perform the operation. For a woman who wishes to continue or resume sexual intercourse, following a vaginal repair, the surgeon will endeavour to ensure that the repair operation is such that it allows for the woman to have sexual intercourse comfortably, once the vaginal walls are healed and she has fully recovered from the operation.

Following 'repair' surgery women may look forward to a better quality of life, without the uncomfortable symptoms of prolapse.

SURGERY FOR STRESS INCONTINENCE

Stress incontinence is leakage of urine when you cough, sneeze or exercise. Special bladder investigations (urodynamics) may be carried out in order to diagnose the type of incontinence problem and determine the best course of treatment. Stress incontinence is particularly common in women and may be the result of factors such as pregnancy and childbirth, being overweight, or menopausal changes.

Before surgery is considered, a course of supervised pelvic floor muscles training of at least three month's duration should be undertaken as a first-line treatment (NICE 2006), from a specialist continence physiotherapist or continence nurse. These need to be practised on a daily and regular basis (see pages 29–31). A high rate of women may get improvement from exercises. If these fail then surgery may be the next step.

TVT (Tension-free vaginal tape) or TOT (Trans Obturator Tape)

TVT/TOT has become the operation of choice for most patients with stress incontinence. There are a wide variety of TVT-like procedures – the name varies according to the company which makes the particular device. The operation may be done as a day-case procedure or may involve an overnight stay in hospital. It has a short recovery period.

The operation takes about thirty minutes and may be carried out under general, spinal or local anaesthetic, and involves placing a permanent tape under the urethra or bladder outlet. This permanent tape provides support to the bladder neck when it is most under strain, i.e. when you laugh, cough, sneeze or exercise, and so prevents leaking of urine.

You may experience some aches and pains in the pubic area following a TVT or on the inside of your thighs after a TOT, although this should settle down over the next few days.

Pelvic floor muscles exercise is recommended after this operation, but always first ask your doctor or physiotherapist when you should start.

Have a rest the first few days you are home; if there is any bleeding, pain or difficulty passing urine, contact the hospital ward or your GP. A urinary infection may occur in a small number of cases but is usually easily treated with antibiotics and increased fluids.

You may shower any time after surgery, however avoid having perfumed baths, for example a bubble bath, until the wounds are fully healed.

The post-operative time is short with most women returning to normal routine within about two weeks.

It is *not* advisable to return to sport, running, the gym, cycling or heavy lifting for about 6–8 weeks.

These precautions are important to allow the wounds to heal and the permanent tape to settle into place. Always ask your doctor if you are uncertain about returning to any specific activity.

TVT/TOT is suitable for most women, even those who have had continence surgery in the past. It is not suitable if you are pregnant. If you want children in the future, you can have a TVT/TOT but may be advised to have a caesarean delivery. It may be combined with vaginal repair surgery, and then aftercare advice would be the same as for vaginal repair (see page 20).

Risk factors in TVT/TOT

Serious complications are rare. Your hospital consultant will explain any possible problems to you. Some women may need to have an indwelling catheter for a few days and occasionally longer until normal bladder function returns. The urinary stream may be slower initially and there may be some urinary urgency.

Colposuspension

Colposuspension used to be the commonest major procedure for stress incontinence and is now much less commonly performed due to the popularity of TVT/TOT. It involves lifting the neck of the bladder into a new and corrected position, thus preventing the loss of urine. It is usually performed through a bikini-line abdominal incision, as for hysterectomy. During the operation a catheter (fine, flexible tube) is inserted into the bladder through the lower abdomen to drain off the urine. You may need to have a catheter for about three or four days, sometimes longer, while you have a bladder retraining programme. This involves clamping the catheter every day to help you to try and pass urine normally. The process is repeated every day until this is achieved and then the catheter is removed. *Drinking adequate fluids is important.*

Risk factors in colposuspension

Serious complications are rare and the operation is generally safe and successful. However, no surgery is without risk and the health care team will discuss this with you.

The health care team are very aware of the risks involved and preventative measures are taken to help minimise all potential risk factors, which in general are very low. The advice in this booklet with regard to recovery following your operation applies equally to hysterectomy, vaginal repair surgery and colposuspension.

PREPARE FOR YOUR OPERATION

General advice

In general, try not to get too tired before admission. It will also be a good idea to plan ahead for when you return home. Try to arrange some help with everyday tasks such as shopping for food and keeping your home in order during your convalescent time. Remember yourself too – plan ahead for any interests you could enjoy during your convalescent period.

It is not wise to bring valuables, jewellery or large amounts of money into hospital. Just have some small change for the telephone and newspapers (although you may be allowed to use a mobile phone). Remember that your concentration is likely to be low after the anaesthetic, so think about bringing something easy to read.

You will be discharged when medical care is no longer necessary, i.e. two to five days after your surgery. Try to arrange some help at home for your convalescence. This may be a time to think about your long-term future, particularly if you have a job which involves heavy lifting. You may wish to discuss this point with the doctors and nurses looking after you, or afterwards with your own doctor.

You may be entitled to sick pay and benefits, so do find out about this from your employer or from the Department for Work and Pensions.

Physical fitness

Your rate of recovery following your operation is likely to be better if you are in reasonably good shape.

Practise getting in and out of bed correctly, as described and illustrated on pages 27–29.

You may find it helpful to practise deep breathing (page 26) and the pelvic floor muscles exercise (pages 29–31).

Smoking

If you do smoke, try not to smoke for at least three days before and after your operation. *This is a good opportunity to give up smoking.* Prior to an anaesthetic it is particularly important to have your lungs free from cigarette smoke. It is also worth remembering that most hospitals operate a no-smoking policy, so you need to be prepared for this.

Diet

Try and eat a healthy diet before going into hospital. If you are over-weight, try to lose a few pounds. (See 'Weight Control and Eating Sensibly', page 35.)

Emotional wellbeing

You may find you are facing all sorts of feelings about your forthcoming surgery, from great relief to sadness or shock. You may be unsure about whether you are making the right decision by going ahead, or you may be worrying about particular issues of concern to you personally. Sometimes it can be difficult to make sense of all these different feelings, and so you may find it helpful to talk them through with someone close to you or with the health professionals looking after you.

Cultural/religious issues

It may be that a woman's role in her culture is dependent on her fertility. This can be especially disconcerting if she is no longer able to fulfil these expectations. Some cultures or religions may have other issues which cause specific concern with regard to this type of surgery. The conflict between beliefs and reality may result in difficult and painful decisions. If this applies to you, do talk about your feelings as this may help you to come to terms with them.

Pre-operative assessment

Most hospitals provide a pre-operative assessment service, which will involve you attending the hospital for an appointment about one to two weeks before you are admitted for your operation. The hospital staff will assess you to check whether you are fit for the operation and various investigations may be carried out, such as blood tests, ECG (heart tracing), blood pressure check, and urine testing. You may get the opportunity then to ask questions and raise any concerns about your hospital stay. You could find it helpful to write a list of questions before your appointment, so that you don't forget what you want to ask.

ADMISSION TO HOSPITAL

You may either be admitted on the day before your operation or on the actual day. On admission, do not hesitate to raise any last-minute worries or anxieties you may have. Remember to tell the hospital staff if you are taking any regular medication, including the contraceptive pill and any alternative medicines. Also mention if you have taken any drugs recently, or have any allergies, whether you have any caps or crowns in your teeth, and whether you require a special diet (for example, diabetic or low fat, etc.).

It is a good idea to find out about ward visiting times before coming into hospital, and also to discourage visitors – other than your close relatives – for the first few days, as they can be very tiring and you will not feel like entertaining!

Pre-operative preparation

To prepare you for your operation you will be told to have nothing to eat or drink for several hours beforehand. The nursing staff will want to ensure that your bowels are empty and may wish to clip or shave hair from your pubic area. You may be fitted with special support ('anti-embolic') stockings, which reduce the risk of thrombosis (blood clots in the blood vessels). Blood and urine samples may be taken and tested, if this has not already been done at your pre-admission appointment.

It is usual to have a bath or shower before going to the operating theatre and you will also be asked to remove contact lenses, false teeth, make-up, nail varnish, jewellery and body piercings.

During the operation

Usually you will have a general anaesthetic for the operation. This means that you will be asleep for the duration of the operation, but you will be closely monitored throughout by the anaesthetist (the doctor who will have put you to sleep for the operation). Sometimes the anaesthetist will decide to use a different form of anaesthetic (regional or epidural anaesthesia). This involves injections which numb a larger or deeper part of the body. You may stay conscious, though free from pain and discomfort. This is usually accompanied by a sedating drug to make you feel relaxed during the procedure. The staff caring for you will be experienced health care professionals who will endeavour to ensure that you are well looked after, that the operation is successful and that any possible risks are kept to a minimum.

Immediate post-operative recovery period

Once the operation has been completed, you will be taken to a recovery area close to the operating theatre, for a short period of time. This could be anything from half an hour up to several hours, depending on your rate of recovery. At first you are likely to feel quite sleepy and may be aware of having an oxygen mask or similar device attached to your face. A health care professional who is experienced in caring for patients following operations will be looking after you, on a one-to-one basis in the recovery area. Once your condition is considered to be stable, you will be transferred to a different, less acute room or ward where you will spend the majority of your recovery time in hospital.

GENERAL CARE AFTER YOUR OPERATION

Pain relief

The degree of pain or discomfort experienced by individuals following surgery varies a great deal. Bruising and soreness around the area of the wound may extend to include the whole genital area following the operation, but usually eases after a few days. Injections or special suppositories (small pellets inserted into your back passage) may be

20

offered initially to relieve pain, then simple pain-killing tablets are usually sufficient to reduce the discomfort.

Patient-controlled analgesia (PCA)

This may be offered after certain operations. A small device is attached to your arm or hand, which enables you to obtain small amounts of pain relief, directly into the bloodstream, as and when you need it. You will be given information about this facility by the hospital staff, if it is appropriate.

Other methods of pain relief

Other methods of pain relief include a local anaesthetic injection administered into the operation site or a system such as the pain-buster post-operative pain relief system, which provides a continuous infusion of local anaesthetic directly into the operation site. Another method of continuous pain relief may be provided by means of an epidural, which is administered via a small tube into the epidural space in your spine.

The first few days following your operation

It will take a day or two for your body to recover from the stress of the operation and the effects of the anaesthetic and any strong pain relief you have had. You will be a little sleepy, will lack energy and may even feel rather sick and dizzy. You may feel vulnerable and restricted at first, but the nursing staff will be there to help you through this initial period. They will provide the care that you need, as well as being there to monitor your recovery closely. However, it won't be long before you are up and about and able to fend for yourself.

Depression, or 'post-op' blues

It is not uncommon to feel emotional or weepy immediately following your operation. Many women experience these feelings, but usually only for a few days. Don't be surprised if these feelings come back when you get home, having left the security of the hospital setting. They are a normal reaction and should pass quickly.

Food and drink

For a few hours or sometimes longer following your operation it may be necessary to give you fluids intravenously (through a drip into a vein – usually in the arm), although you should soon be eating and drinking normally. You may be advised to drink plenty of fluids following your operation, once this is permitted. Until then, do ask for a mouthwash if your mouth feels dry. Some people feel sick following an operation. If you do, make sure you let the medical or nursing staff know, as they can give you some medicines to help relieve this feeling.

Bladder care in hospital after hysterectomy and vaginal repair *(for colposuspension see page 16–17)*

Everyone differs as to when their normal bladder function is restored. Passing urine is usually not a problem, although the flow can sometimes be slow at first or even completely obstructed, due to bruising and also due to the reaction of some of the drugs that are used during and immediately after the operation. You should be able to use a commode beside the bed or to walk to the toilet fairly soon after the operation, but sometimes a catheter (a thin flexible tube) may be inserted into the bladder to drain the urine away. This may be removed a day or so after the operation or it may be left in place a few days longer, in order to rest the repaired tissues. This causes very little discomfort and the bag containing the urine can be placed in a discreet position. Drinking adequate fluids after the operation will help to prevent any urinary infections – this is particularly important if a catheter is in place. Occasionally it may be necessary to go home with a catheter for a few days and then to return for a day to have it removed and check that you can pass urine successfully.

Bowels and wind

It is quite usual not to have a bowel motion for the first three or four days after the operation, as the nurses will have ensured that your bowels are empty beforehand. Tell the staff if you have not had your bowels open by the day before you go home. You may need to be given a laxative, because straining should be avoided. You may find that it helps to support the area between your legs just in front of your back passage with a pad when passing a bowel motion or wind.

To empty your bowels and bladder adopt the correct position (Figure 9):

Sit on the toilet with your legs apart, lean forward resting your elbows on your knees, raise up on your toes so that your knees are higher than your hips, keep your back straight and relax your tummy muscles as you empty your bowels and bladder. Remember not to strain, to avoid holding your breath, and to take your time. At home you could put your feet up on a low block about the height of two telephone directories, or 10–15 cm. Use this pattern after your surgery and continue with it for the rest of your life.

Figure 9   *The correct position for emptying the bowels and bladder.*

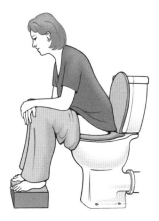

If constipation is a problem when you go home, see the advice on page 36.

Wind may be a real problem and can be very uncomfortable. Gently walking around and changing your position regularly may be helpful. It may also help to do the pelvic tilting or the knee rolling exercises described on pages 32–33. The nursing staff can advise on relieving the discomfort, possibly by giving you a warm peppermint-type 'cocktail' or with simple painkillers. Some women experience pain in the right shoulder area. This is a 'referred' pain caused by the accumulation of wind in the abdomen. A few deep breaths in and out may help to relieve it. *Always tell the nursing staff if you have shoulder pain.*

Wound care

A thin drainage tube may be left in place following surgery to remove any excess fluid collecting beneath the wound. The drained fluid (which is likely to be bloodstained) runs into a small bottle or bag. The tube is removed after a day or two, depending on how much drainage there is.

23

Stitches

When an abdominal operation is carried out, the cut on the abdomen is closed using clips or stitches which are removed following the operation. Alternatively, some surgeons use stitches made of a dissolvable material, which do not need to be removed and which will dissolve completely when the area is healed. The stitches in the vagina are also soluble. Abdominal stitches and clips, which are not dissolvable, are normally removed between the fourth and sixth day after the operation; this should not be a painful procedure. The nurses caring for you during your hospital stay can tell you which sort of stitches or clips have been used. Numbness or a loss of sensation to touch may be experienced afterwards in the area around the scar tissue. The scar will at first be a red line, which may feel a little lumpy, and there may be some pulling as it heals. This will gradually fade until about a year later, when it will look like a thin white line.

The healing appears rapid on the outside, but it must be remembered that all the many layers of muscle and tissue have to heal internally and this takes much longer.

Hygiene

A daily bath or shower will be encouraged following the operation. If you have abdominal stitches you must dry this area until they dissolve or are removed.

Vaginal bleeding or discharge

A slight vaginal discharge is normal for up to six weeks following hysterectomy or repair. It is possible for the discharge to contain threads from dissolving internal vaginal stitches. If the discharge becomes bright red, heavy or with clots, or if it becomes thicker and smells offensive, please rest and *seek medical advice at once*. Only use sanitary pads and change them regularly. *Never* use tampons because of the possibility of introducing infection into the vagina.

Rest

Rest is essential as part of the healing process, both during the day as well as at night. Try to have at least one hour's rest during the day. Lie with pillows under your head but otherwise flat, either on your back or side, whichever is more comfortable. You may find that lying on your side with your knees bent up, or leaning on a pillow cuddled to your tummy, will be helpful. After vaginal surgery you may also find that lying face down with a pillow at waist level is comfortable and rests your back. Remember to keep visitors to a minimum during the first few days, as they can be quite exhausting.

Circulation, and prevention of thrombosis

You may be asked to wear special stockings, called 'anti-embolic stockings', for a while, and possibly after going home, to help prevent the risk of thrombosis (blood clots in your blood vessels). These may feel rather hot but it is important that they should be worn as advised. Anticoagulant (blood-thinning) injections may be given until you are up and moving freely, also to prevent thrombosis. You can also help yourself with some simple leg exercises.

Leg exercises

Do the following to improve the circulation in your legs: (i) with your knees straight, bend your feet up and down at the ankle, firmly and quickly several times each hour (Figure 10); and (ii) gently bend and stretch your legs one at a time. Do these exercises in bed and also when you are sitting in a chair. When sitting, avoid pressure on the back of your knees by using a footstool if necessary. Do not sit with your legs or ankles crossed, as this restricts the circulation.

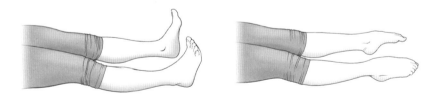

Figure 10   *To improve circulation: (a) legs straight; (b) bend and stretch ankles.*

Also, (iii) with your legs straight, tighten the strong muscles on the front of the thigh by pressing the knee back against the bed while pointing your toes towards the ceiling; hold for a few seconds and let go.

25

Do this as often as possible, either sitting in a chair or standing. This will not only improve the circulation, but will help to prevent your legs feeling 'wobbly' or weak in the early days after your operation. However, it is important for you to be walking about as soon as possible after your operation.

Initially after surgery it is quite safe to move around in bed to make yourself comfortable, and this also helps improve your circulation. There is no danger of bursting your stitches.

Deep breathing

This helps to reduce the effect of the anaesthetic. Start as soon as you wake up. Sit up in bed, supported by pillows, knees bent up, feet flat on the bed. Take a slow deep breath in, fill your lungs with air, hold your breath for the count of two, and sigh the breath out.

Do this three or four times every hour. Remember also to do this breathing exercise when you are sitting out of bed in a chair. It may help to relieve nausea (feelings of sickness) and aid relaxation.

Huffing

Take a deep breath in, then do a short sharp breath out. Do this several times. This breathing technique may help to clear any mucus from your chest.

Coughing

Most people feel the need to cough after an anaeshetic. It is quite safe – the stitches will not burst, and it will hurt less if you do it properly. Use the same sitting position as for deep breathing. If you have had an abdominal incision, put your hands or forearms over the wound, or cuddle a pillow to your tummy (Figure 11); take a deep breath in and then cough, spitting any mucus out. Repeat as you feel it necessary.

If you have had surgery through your vagina, put your hand over your sanitary pad, hold firmly, and cough, spitting any mucus out into a tissue or container. Do this three or four times until your chest feels clear.

After the anaesthetic you may have a sore throat for a few days, which is quite normal, and can be relieved by medication if required.

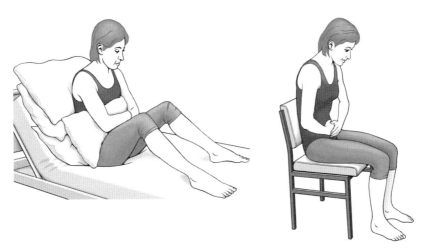

Figure 11   *Coughing, showing position of hands, with or without a pillow:*
(a) in bed; (b) sitting in a chair.

Back care in bed

When sitting up in bed, make sure you have a pillow in the middle
of your lower back to maintain the normal hollow at waist level.

As already mentioned, lie flat at night with pillows under your
head, either on your back or side – whichever you find more
comfortable.

Turning over in bed

Draw in your lower tummy very gently. Bend your knees up, keeping
them pressed together. Roll over with shoulders and knees in line, so
that you do not twist. Think of your body as a log of wood – turning in
this way protects the wound and is less painful.

Getting out of bed

On the first day after your operation you usually sit out in a chair for
a short time – this will help your circulation following surgery, particularly as you will be less mobile than usual.

Getting out of bed correctly will put less strain on your operation site.
Draw in your lower tummy very gently. Bend your knees up, roll onto
your side keeping your knees together, push yourself up into a sitting

position with your hands, allowing your legs to swing down to the floor (Figure 12). Reverse this process to get back into bed.

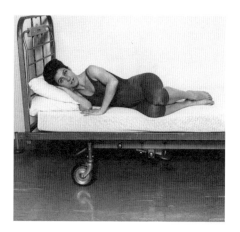
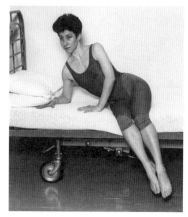

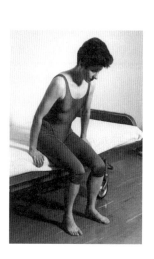
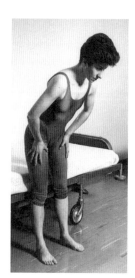
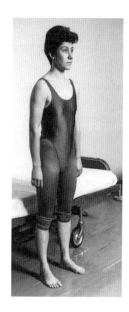

Figure 12   *Getting out of bed: (a) Draw in lower tummy very gently, roll to side, knees together, note position of hands (see 'Turning over in Bed'); (b) Swing legs down, keeping knees bent, and push up with hands to sitting position; (c) Sit on side of bed, feet apart and flat on floor; (d) Lean forward, straighten knees, and stand up; (e) Stand up straight before beginning to walk.*

Gradually, stand up straight, wait for a few seconds to get used to your upright position, and then begin to walk. Do not be anxious about standing up straight, as this will be beneficial for you. When you first get out of bed you may feel a little unsteady on your feet at first, so ask for help if you need it.

Posture

Remember – 'stand tall' and 'walk tall'. Always stand up straight and pull your tummy muscles in. This will support your back – and if you have abdominal stitches it will not interfere with their healing. This is a good pattern for the rest of your life.

EXERCISES AFTER YOUR OPERATION

The pelvic floor muscles

Exercising your pelvic floor muscles is *essential*. These muscles form a sling or 'hammock' which passes from the pubic bones at the front of the pelvis to the tailbone (coccyx) at the back, and forms the floor to the pelvis. This sling also loops round the urinary passage (urethra), the vagina (birth canal), and the back passage (anus) and as a result helps to control these outlets from the pelvic organs (see Figure 3, page 3).

It is important to keep this sling of muscles healthy and strong. This enables them to support the abdominal organs efficiently, helping to prevent prolapse. The pelvic floor muscles also help control the function of the bladder and bowel and so prevent the symptoms of urinary and bowel incontinence. This may present as leaks of urine on sudden movement – for example, on coughing or laughing, or at an exercise class or running for a bus. Weakness may also result in reduced sexual satisfaction.

These muscles may become weakened after pregnancy and child-birth, or as a result of ageing, being overweight, or decreased levels of physical activity.

Pelvic floor exercises are therefore very important, especially if you have these problems now, or else to prevent problems later.

The pelvic floor muscles exercise

Before your operation it will have been beneficial for you to practise this exercise. *After your operation check first with your doctor or physiotherapist how soon you may start again.* As a general rule you can begin after your catheter has been removed. The exercise should be done in different positions – lying, sitting or standing – with your legs slightly apart.

Tighten up round your back passage as if to stop passing wind, and at the same time tighten up round your front passage as if to stop a leak of urine. The feeling is one of squeeze and lift. As you contract your pelvic floor muscles you may feel your lower abdomen drawing in gently – this is quite normal. Remember to keep breathing, and keep your spine straight.

Once you can do this basic exercise you will need to start a simple exercise programme. The aim is to build up the strength of the muscles by increasing the length of time you hold the contraction and the number of times you do it.

The exercise programme:
1) Tighten your pelvic floor muscles as described and try to hold this contraction for as many seconds as you can, gradually increasing over the weeks up to a maximum hold of 10 seconds.
2) Repeat the exercise as many times as you can, resting briefly (for example, a count of 5 seconds) between contractions. The pelvic floor muscles tire easily, so stop when you find your ability to hold is becoming weaker. Gradually increase to a maximum of 10 as your muscles become stronger.
3) Now add a fast one-second *squeeze and let go*, and try to repeat this as many times as you can, up to a maximum of ten times. Rest briefly between contractions. Make these short contractions as strong as possible.
4) Remember not to hold your breath.

This exercise programme should be repeated at three times a day. When you start you may only be able to hold a contraction for two or three seconds and repeat it two or three times, with the same number of short quick contractions. Over the next few weeks you should be able to gradually increase the length of the 'hold' time of the contraction and the number of repetitions you can do, as your muscles build up in strength.

These exercises will help to control leaks of urine as well as a whole range of symptoms such as 'urgency' (a need to rush to the toilet) and 'frequency' (a need to pass urine very often during the day). These problems occasionally arise after surgery.

Always remember to tighten your pelvic floor muscles when you lift, push, pull, sneeze, cough or exercise. This is why fast one-second squeezes are useful, so that you can train the muscles to react strongly and quickly when necessary.

Try to get into the habit of doing the pelvic floor muscles exercise as described, daily and regularly. If you think you are likely to forget, associate the exercise routine with an everyday activity such as making a cup of tea, waiting for a bus or train, queuing at a checkout or watching TV adverts.

And *remember* – continue to do this pelvic floor muscles exercise always – for the rest of your life!

The abdominal muscles

The abdominal (tummy) muscles form an elastic corset which acts as a brace to your spine and protects you from back pain. Fat is attracted to the tissues between the abdominal muscle layers and so attention to diet is important.

The next three exercises are of particular value following abdominal surgery. Do not worry if you find them difficult at first – they will become easier with each day – and should not cause pain or discomfort.

Abdominal hollowing exercise (Figure 13)

This exercise may be started in the first few days following surgery. Work the deep muscles first – these are very important as they help to stabilise the spine and pelvis, and will also help to flatten your tummy.

You may do the exercise in any comfortable position – lying on your back or side with your knees bent up, sitting up in bed, or in a chair.

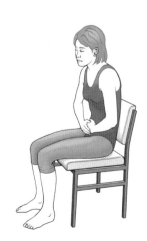

Figure 13   *Abdominal hollowing exercise.*

31

Keeping your back straight, place one hand on the lower part of your abdomen, making sure your tummy muscles are relaxed. Take a breath in, and as you breathe out gently draw in the lower part of your tummy away from your hand and towards your spine. Try to hold for a count of five (5 seconds) while continuing to breathe normally. You may find you can pull up your pelvic floor muscles at the same time, but remember not to move your back.

Do this exercise four or five times at first, gradually building up to ten times – with a few seconds rest between each one. Repeat three times a day, gradually increasing the hold time to 10-15 seconds.

This is another exercise to do for the rest of your life. When you get home try to get into the habit of doing it during everyday activities such as standing and walking. Try doing it in bed, at night, lying on your side with your knees bent up.

Once you can do the abdominal hollowing exercise, you can progress to the pelvic tilting and knee rolling exercises.

Pelvic tilting (Figure 14)

Lie on your back, one pillow under your head, knees bent up, feet on the bed. *Do the abdominal hollowing exercise, tighten your pelvic floor, tilt your bottom upwards slightly and try to press the middle of your back flat against the mattress. Hold for the count of five, then relax. Do not hold your breath and do not press down on your feet.* Repeat six times, at least three times daily. Try this pelvic tilting movement in a sitting position and also in standing and walking, to correct your posture. This exercise should ease backache and help to reduce flatulence.

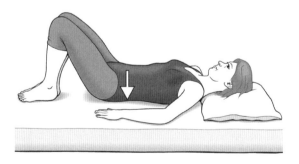

Figure 14 *Pelvic tilting.*

Knee rolling (or tick-tock exercise) (Figure 15)

Lie on your back with your knees bent up, feet on the bed, one pillow under your head. *Start once again with the abdominal hollowing exercise. As you breathe out, move both knees to the left in a small controlled movement and, as you breathe in, return to the starting position. Remember not to hold your breath.*

Figure 15   *Knee rolling.*

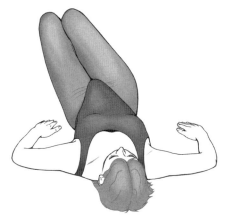

Repeat to the right.
Do not move your back and remember not to hold your breath.
Repeat six times, three times daily.
This exercise may also relieve flatulence.

As you recover, continue with the above exercises for at least six weeks.

AFTER LEAVING HOSPITAL

Hysterectomy, vaginal repair and colposuspension can all involve fairly extensive internal surgery. Although an external scar is likely to heal quickly – usually within a week – the internal healing process takes considerably longer.

The majority of patients are well enough to leave hospital a few days after their operation. This varies according to your individual rate of recovery, the advice of the hospital staff and the method and extent of the surgery performed.

The recovery time is very important. Resting and following advice carefully will ensure that the tissues heal correctly – and *remember* that the success of your operation depends on this.

Rest and exercise

When you go home you will need at least a week's extended 'hospital' care. That means resting, getting up when you want to, relaxing and – of course – continuing with the exercises.

Try to avoid standing still for more than a few minutes at a time. If you keep your legs moving it will help your circulation. It is sensible to sit in a comfortable chair which is not too low, with armrests, when you first get home.

The convalescent period

The convalescent period is a very important time and your body must be given time to heal. Your progress is likely to happen in stages and is a unique experience for each individual woman. A successful recovery depends very much on the extent of your surgery, your general health prior to surgery, how you felt about having the operation, your domestic situation, the information, verbal and written, that you have received, and a careful lifestyle during your convalescence.

Fatigue

You may find you tire easily. Don't feel anxious if you find this tiredness continues for some weeks. The return to normal life following any major operation takes time and is a gradual process. In general, do what you feel you sensibly can, but don't push yourself too hard too soon! Don't persist with any activity that you can't achieve easily. Only you know how much you can do, and remember that everyone is individual. You will gain strength gradually, so if you find the guidelines for activity and exercise suggested in this booklet are difficult to achieve, give yourself an extra day or two and then try again. Don't feel a failure because you know of others who have recovered more quickly. Remember, always extend activities slowly and at the pace your body dictates.

Vulnerability

Women may also feel emotionally vulnerable for a while – it is reassuring to know that this is a common experience. Your morale will improve as your recovery progresses. The help and understanding of family and friends, if you are fortunate enough to have this support, can be invaluable at this time.

Concentration

Many women find their ability to concentrate is affected following surgery for a variable length of time, so this may influence your normal activities of daily living.

Personal cleanliness

It is important to continue to have a daily bath or shower once you have left hospital (unless you have been specifically told not to). It may be a good idea to bath when someone else is at home in case you have problems getting out of the bath at first. Use a non-slip mat if you have a shower and pay special attention to cleaning the genital area. Try to wear cotton pants that sit well above the wound – this will be more comfortable and also prevent unnecessary touching of the area and so prevent infection.

Weight control and eating sensibly

There is no reason why you should gain weight following a hysterectomy. If you follow the dietary advice which follows and take gradually increased regular exercise, you should stay at your normal weight. Being overweight can put extra pressure on the bladder too, so try and stay within healthy guidelines for your height. Ask the nursing staff about this, or else you should be able to get this information at your local surgery.

A well-balanced nutritious diet containing a high fibre content is essential to avoid constipation. Eat plenty of fresh fruit, salads, green vegetables and wholemeal bread. Try to make sure you get enough food that contains protein, such as meat, eggs, and fish, or pulses (peas, beans, lentils) if you are a vegetarian. Avoid fried and stodgy foods, cakes, pastries, sweets and chocolate. Drink plenty of fluids – at least one and a half to two litres a day.

Constipation

This is frequently a problem following pelvic surgery and may result from having a diet low in roughage and fluids, and also lack of exercise. It is important to use the correct position for emptying your bowels (see 'Bowels and Wind', pages 22–23) and do remember that the pelvic floor muscles exercise will be helping to give better bowel control as well. Straining to pass a motion can be harmful and should be avoided. If a laxative is required, a mild remedy may be recommended by a pharmacist or your doctor.

Urinary problems

Slight discomfort and difficulties with bladder function are sometimes experienced by a small number of women following surgery, but such problems are usually temporary and should settle down fairly soon after you go home. Burning pain when you pass urine may indicate a urinary infection, and medical advice should be sought.

If urgency occurs (an immediate need to pass urine), do your best to keep calm, breathe gently, stand still or sit on a firm chair or stool, and distract your thoughts by thinking of something else such as reciting the words of a song or counting, and do your pelvic floor muscles exercise. When the desire to pass urine stops, which may take about 10-15 seconds, then walk to the toilet. But you should also consult your doctor, and take note of the following bladder care advice.

Bladder care at home

When you get home try and continue to use good bladder habits. As we have said, drink one and a half to two litres of fluid a day (water is best). Avoid going to the toilet 'just in case' – only empty your bladder when you need to. Limit your caffeine intake – found in coffee and tea (as well as cola drinks and chocolate) – as it may irritate your bladder; it may be helpful to swap to a decaffeinated brand. When you pass urine take your time and make sure your bladder is completely empty, without straining. This will reduce the risk of cystitis and infection. Adopt the correct position (page 23), and continue to do your pelvic floor muscles exercise.

Stairs

It is quite safe to go up and down stairs after you have been discharged from hospital, but always remember to hold on to the handrail.

Housework

Have a rest for the first few days you are home. However, you can make a cup of tea, help with washing up, dusting and easy household jobs, etc. Reduce your standing. Sit on a stool or chair wherever possible.

About three to four weeks after your operation you can gradually start to do more household jobs, such as cooking and ironing and using a mop or *lightweight* vacuum cleaner (Figure 16), with the exception of work involving heavy lifting or prolonged standing.

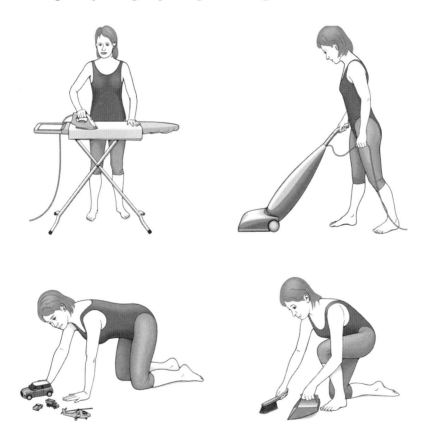

Figure 16 *Housework: (a) Ironing – note feet apart and correct height of ironing board to keep back straight; (b) Hoovering and mopping – note feet apart and back straight; (c) Cleaning the floor, picking up toys or weeding; (d) Using a dustpan and brush.*

Lifting

For the first four weeks reduce lifting whenever possible to allow the tissues to heal correctly and avoid future damage. As a guide, do not lift more than a full kettle of water or its equivalent, i.e. 3–4 kg. Heavy lifting or moving furniture should not be attempted until *at least* three months after surgery. The ideal situation would be to avoid such unnecessary heavy activities for the rest of your life, but obviously this is not always realistic. This will also help to ensure that the benefits of your surgery last longer.

Remember: When you do lift, do it correctly. With your feet placed apart in the walking position, bend your knees, back straight, gently pull in your lower tummy and tighten your pelvic floor muscles, hold the object to be lifted or carried close to you, and lift by straightening your knees (Figure 17).

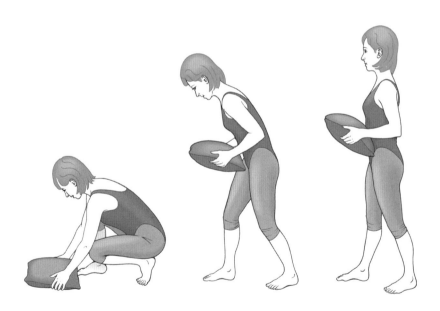

Figure 17   *How to lift correctly: (a) Bend knees, back straight, pull lower tummy in, tighten pelvic floor muscles, hold object to be lifted close to you; (b) Lift by straightening your knees; (c) Back straight, holding object close to you.*

Walking

Walking is the perfect exercise. When you go home you should aim for a ten-minute walk daily, gradually increasing to a 30–45 minute walk by four weeks, or two short walks, if you prefer. But remember – only walk the distance you can achieve comfortably.

Driving

To get into a car comfortably, stand with the back of your legs close to the car seat, bend forwards from the hips, bend your knees and sit backwards into the car seat using your hands on the car door frame to steady yourself. Pull in your tummy muscles and lift first one leg and then the other slowly into the car. Remember – do not twist your back. Get out of the car in the same way, but always stand up straight before walking away.

It is usually safe to drive the car about three to four weeks following surgery, although after any operation this will depend on your confidence and concentration, and also on your ability to do an emergency stop. But – check first that your car insurance policy does not have an exclusion or impose special conditions relating to major surgery.

Back to work

Your own doctor will advise you when to return to work. It may be any time between six and twelve weeks, depending on the type of work involved, and of course the extent of your surgery and the rate of your recovery. However, it is generally accepted that employers should be prepared to allow up to three months sick leave for these operations. Initially, part-time or flexi-hours may have to be negotiated. Follow the advice of your surgeon/doctor with regard to resuming any job where heavy lifting is involved. Travel to and from work may also need to be reassessed – a door-to-door lift by car being preferable to the stresses of travel by public transport, if at all possible. Consider walking to work if this is an option. Any plans for long-distance travel should be discussed with your doctor.

It may be necessary to reassess your working conditions, to enable you to sit rather than stand for long periods, and if need be request a more suitable chair. If you have a job which involves sitting for long periods, perhaps using a computer, do make sure that your back is well supported, that your feet can rest comfortably on the floor, and that the computer is positioned so that you do not need to twist your back (Figure 18). If the chair is too high, ask for a stool to rest your feet on. If you find it helps, use a small pillow to support the natural curve of your lower back, and remember to get up and walk around for a few minutes every now and then.

Employers and work colleagues, particularly males, may not always appreciate the implications of your recent surgery and may need educating! You may also need to be assertive to ensure your future health and full recovery – if necessary supported by a letter from your doctor. Try to discuss your operation and its implications with your manager/boss before your operation.

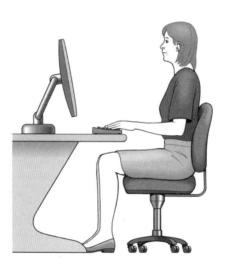

Figure 18   *Sitting at a desk: back supported, feet flat on floor.*

Travel and holidays

You might wish to avoid long car, coach, bus or train journeys for a few weeks following your operation, as you may feel tired and uncomfortable at this early stage. Also, you are best advised not to arrange to take a holiday until you feel well enough, especially if this involves a long journey or foreign travel. If you are planning an air flight, particularly long-haul, you need to seek the advice of your doctor and travel insurance company in advance.

Sport and other activities

The rate of recovery from surgery varies for everyone. As a guide it should be safe to start gentle exercise about six to eight weeks after the operation, following the approval of the doctor at your post-operative check. Exercise classes at a beginner's standard or Pilates mat work Level 1, if these are available at a local leisure centre, or a specially tailored training programme by a qualified instructor, would be a good way to begin a gradual return to fitness. It is important to follow the pace your body dictates and not to push yourself beyond your ability to cope comfortably. A gentle return is essential.

Only begin with those activities that can be stopped at any point when you feel tired.

Gentle swimming for pleasure can usually be started after about a month, providing any discharge has stopped. At first choose a quiet time when there are few people in the pool.

It is advisable not to return to competitive sports or high-impact aerobics for three months after surgery, following a gradual build-up to fitness.

Digging or any heavy garden work which involves lifting must not be attempted until at least twelve weeks following surgery, and then only with caution.

If there are any doubts or special circumstances, ask your doctor for advice.

Warning: Never try to do the following while lying on your back: (i) lifting both legs together while straight; and (ii) 'sit-ups' with legs straight.

Sexual activity

There are a lot of misconceptions and 'old wives' tales' about a woman's sexual life following hysterectomy. Women need love and affection at this time and enjoy the close physical contact of cuddling and touching. They and their partners often request specific advice about resuming sexual intercourse. If the opportunity exists, it may be helpful for you and your partner to discuss the operation with a health professional beforehand.

Many women feel tired and indifferent to sex after hysterectomy and their interest may only return gradually. This may involve the need for your confidence as a woman to be restored, regardless of whether you have a womb or not.

In order to understand exactly what advice we give and why, it is important first of all to understand a little of the female anatomy and how the reproductive organs are affected during the operation (see Figures 1, 2, 3 and 4).

The vagina is just a passage into which protrudes the cervix (entrance to the womb). As already described, during hysterectomy the womb and usually the cervix as well are removed. This obviously involves some surgery and repair by stitching to the far end of the vagina. Initially, this shortens the passage very slightly, but as the vagina is lined with folds of stretchy skin, this should create no problem when sexual intercourse is resumed. This depends very much on the extent of the vaginal surgery, the rate of healing and the couple's own preference.

Many women prefer to wait until after the post-operative check (usually about six weeks) to be sure the area is completely healed. This is because sexual arousal (not only intercourse) tends to have a stretching effect on the vagina and could interfere with the healing process. Once this area is completely healed, sexual activity may be resumed.

Because the size and angle of the vagina may have been altered slightly, it may be wise to try out different positions for intercourse to find how you are most comfortable.

Obviously, your sexual partner should be gentle at first. It may also help considerably to use a proprietary lubricant (obtainable from any chemist). This is because the vagina may not produce enough natural lubrication while you are tense or apprehensive about resuming sexual activity. Your partner may feel apprehensive at first, so do try and talk about your fears and anxieties about sex after your surgery.

Most women find it reassuring to know that their own sexual response should be very little changed by the operation, since the external reproductive organs are unaltered. If a climax is normally experienced, this will still be possible. Many women find that their sexual response actually improves, as the physical problems they were experiencing prior to surgery have been removed, along with the risk of pregnancy.

SMEAR TESTS

Women who have undergone a hysterectomy frequently enquire about continuing with 'smear tests'. Where the womb, including the cervix, has been removed, *cervical* smears are no longer possible or necessary.

Where a sub-total hysterectomy has been performed, the cervix remains and smears should continue to be taken. If the womb has been removed because of abnormal cervical smears or cancer, the consultant may wish to continue to observe and take occasional smears from the 'vaginal vault' – the deepest part of the vagina.

THE MENOPAUSE

Many women undergoing hysterectomy and/or vaginal repair ask questions about the menopause, and they may also require information regarding hormone replacement therapy.

The word 'menopause' really means 'last period', but we use it to describe the changes which happen to a woman's body around this time of life, due to the reduction in the activity of the ovaries. The menopause is a natural process that usually occurs at about the age of fifty, but which can happen earlier and later than this. There is often a familial tendency – mother and daughter frequently following a similar menopausal pattern.

Menopausal symptoms are caused by a decrease in the hormone levels produced by the ovaries as they cease to function. These symptoms can also result from the surgical removal of both ovaries which sometimes accompanies hysterectomy (see Figures 1 and 2). The fall in production of these hormones – oestrogen and progesterone – can affect the body in the following areas:

Firstly, the muscles and nerves which control the blood vessels – this may produce the hot flushes, night sweats, palpitations and headaches which some menopausal women experience to a varying degree.

For those women who have *not* undergone a hysterectomy, periods become irregular and eventually cease altogether. Many women welcome the end to a monthly inconvenience, enjoying the freedom from discomfort, bleeding and the expense of purchasing sanitary protection. Vaginal dryness may be experienced, so that sexual intercourse without additional lubrication becomes uncomfortable – and consequently the desire to make love may lessen.

The skin, hair and bones can also be influenced by these hormonal changes – the skin becoming dryer, hair less greasy, thinning and changing in texture. Bones may gradually lose their density, become more brittle and so break more easily. The areas most vulnerable are the hip, spine and wrist. This condition is called osteoporosis and can be greatly helped by appropriate medication, including HRT (see next section), although a calcium-rich diet and regular exercise are also thought to be of great value.

The degree to which each individual woman is affected by these changes, and the time taken in passing through the menopause, varies enormously, with the majority of women experiencing very little discomfort. It is helpful at this time to choose cotton rather than synthetic materials – particularly underwear, nightwear, and bed linen. Light layers of clothing which are easily removed and replaced are more comfortable than thick heavy garments. Tepid rather than hot showers and baths are preferable. Indeed it may temporarily be best to avoid any situations which are hot, airless or crowded.

Additional 'self-help' measures may help to lessen menopausal symptoms. A sensible life style including regular exercise has already been mentioned, and practising relaxation may also be beneficial. Find time to follow your own interests. A well-balanced nutritious diet including particularly the foods rich in calcium, i.e. milk, cheese etc, is also thought to be helpful at this time.

Some women, however, find the menopause a very difficult and lengthy process, with both physical and psychological problems to overcome. For example, coping with hot flushes, sweats and sexual discomfort, and psychological symptoms such as depression, sleeplessness, loss of energy or confidence, and irritability. Where menopausal symptoms are causing severe discomfort, or affecting family relationships or work ability, the situation may be improved by sympathetic professional counselling, understanding family support, and possibly hormone replacement therapy. A number of areas also offer specialist menopause advice, and in some places specialist menopause clinics are available.

HORMONE REPLACEMENT THERAPY (HRT)

If the ovaries are *both* removed, the doctor may advise replacing artificially the hormones that the ovaries normally produce. HRT may also be prescribed to help relieve symptoms experienced when undergoing a natural menopause. In the long term, women's bodies change as a result of oestrogen deficiency and it is possible that many body systems are affected. HRT also comes with certain risks which you should be aware of, so make sure you discuss these, in depth, with the health care team looking after you or with your GP.

HRT is most commonly given in the form of tablets taken daily or as instructed. The tablets may be supplied in a 'calendar' pack. Women may need reassurance about any risks involved in taking HRT, especially if they have other risk factors, such as previous deep vein thrombosis (DVT).

HRT is also available in the form of 'patches' which enable the hormone to be absorbed through the skin. These are small hormone-impregnated discs, one of which is applied to the skin below the waist – usually the outer thigh or buttock – and changed twice a week. They are not disturbed by baths or showers and are a convenient form of HRT, although some women experience a local skin reaction and irritation caused by the patch adhesive. Local application in the form of skin gels or a nasal spray may also be prescribed.

Sometimes HRT is administered in the form of a 'slow release' implant placed under the skin (usually of the abdominal wall or buttock) and renewed approximately every six months.

Women who have not had a hysterectomy may continue to have a monthly bleed while taking HRT (depending on the medication pre-scribed). The length of time for which HRT will be prescribed depends upon the needs of each individual. There does not appear to be an absolute time limit for taking HRT – most women continue with it for approximately two or three years. Women who have undergone a premature menopause have different risks and it is generally recom-mended that they should continue with it at least until the age of 50. Be sure to seek advice about continuing HRT from your doctor.

Alternatives to HRT

For women who are advised not to take HRT or who would prefer not to take it, there are some alternative treatments available.

Conventional drug treatments may help alleviate individual symp-toms, such as Clonidine for relief of hot flushes and vaginal lubricants for relief of vaginal symptoms. Dietary supplements, such as Vitamin B6, Vitamin E, Oil of Evening Primrose and other supplements con-taining minerals such as magnesium, zinc and potassium, may be useful for reducing menopausal symptoms.

There are a large number of alternative therapies currently being used to help women with the menopause. If you wish to consider any of these alternatives, it is important that you find out as much as possible about them before committing yourself to something that may not be suitable for you personally or which may be unsafe. Make sure you do your homework first! Currently there is limited knowledge of these preparations and some of them can interact with other medications you may be taking.

IN CONCLUSION

Your operation should remove the cause of some miserable, painful, uncomfortable and debilitating symptoms. By giving full and accurate information on the surgery and its effect, and thus alleviating much of the anxiety associated with the operation, we hope this booklet will enable you to look forward to a new lease of life.

However, every woman is individual and it is important that you should ask for a full explanation of the diagnosis or suggested surgery in your own particular case. Do not be afraid to ask questions of your consultant, the hospital medical, nursing or physiotherapy staff, or your own GP or practice nurse. By fully understanding your own problem, unnecessary anxiety will be prevented and you will make a speedier and more confident recovery.

USEFUL SOURCES OF INFORMATION

Association of Chartered Physiotherapists in Women's Health. c/o The Chartered Society of Physiotherapy, 14 Bedford Row, London WC1R 4ED. Tel: 020 7306 6666, Mon–Fri 9am–5pm. www.acpwh.org.uk

Bladder & Bowel Foundation, SATRA Innovation Park, Rockingham Road, Kettering NN16 9JH. Tel: 01536 533255; Fax: 0870 770 3249. info@bladderandbowelfoundation.org

British Association for Counselling & Psychotherapy, BACP House, 15 St John's Business Park, Lutterworth LE17 4HB. Tel: 01455 883300; Fax: 01455 550243; Minicom: 01455 550307

The British Menopause Society. www.thebms.org.uk

Cancerbackup, Macmillan Cancer Support, 3 Bath Place, Rivington Street, London EC2A 3JR. Tel: 020 7696 9003, Mon-Fri 9am-noon and 2pm-4.45pm; Fax: 020 7696 9002; Cancer information helpline (UK only): 0808 800 1234 (freephone), 020 7739 2280 (standard rate). Lines staffed by cancer specialist nurses, Mon–Fri 9am–8pm.

Cancerbackup Scotland, Suite 2, 3rd Floor, Cranston House, 104/114 Argyle Street, Glasgow G2 8BH. Tel: 0141 223 7676; Helpline: 0808 800 1234 (freephone) 9am–8pm.

Endometriosis UK, 50 Westminster Palace Gardens, Artillery Row, London SW1P 1RR. Helpline: 0808 808 2227; Tel: 020 7222 2781; Fax: 020 7222 2786. www.endometriosis-uk.org

Family Planning Association (fpa), 50 Featherstone Street, London EC1Y 8QU. Tel: 020 7608 5240; Helpline: 0845 122 8690, Mon–Fri 9am–6pm; Fax: 0845 123 2349. www.fpa.org.uk

Hysterectomy Association. www.hysterectomy-association.org.uk

Hysterectomy Support Network, 3 Lynne Close, Green Street Green, Orpington, Kent BR6 6BS.

Menopause Facts. www.menopausefacts.co.uk

www.menopausematters.co.uk

National Osteoporosis Society, Camerton, Bath BA2 0PJ. Tel: 01761 471771, 0845 130 3076, Mon-Thurs 9am-4.30pm, Fri 9am-4pm. info@nos.org.uk

The Patients Association, PO Box 935, Harrow HA1 3YJ. Tel: 020 8423 9111; Helpline: 0845 608 4455; Fax: 020 8423 9119. www. patients-association.com

Women's Health Concern, 4-6 Eton Place, Marlow, Buckinghamshire SL7 2QA. Tel: 01628 478 473; Fax: 01628 482 743. www.womens-health-concern.org.uk

Alternative therapies

British Acupuncture Council, 63 Jeddo Road, London W12 9HQ. Tel: 020 8735 0400; Fax: 020 8735 0404. www.acupuncture.org.uk

British Complementary Medical Association, PO Box 2074, Seaford BN25 1HQ. Tel: 0845 5977; Fax: 0845 345 5978. www.bcma.co.uk

British Homeopathic Association, 29 Park Street West, Luton LU1 3BE. Tel: 0870 444 3950; Fax: 0870 444 3960. www.trusthomeopathy.org

Register of Qualified Aromatherapists, PO Box 3431, Danbury, Chelmsford CM3 4UA. Tel: 01245 227957; Fax: 01245 222152. admin@rqa-uk.org

ADDITIONAL READING

Bowel Control: Information and Practical Advice, Christine Norton & Michael A. Kamm. Beaconsfield Publishers

Cruising through the Menopause, Maryon Stewart. Random House

Hysterectomy: the Woman's View, Anne Dickson & Nikki Henriques. Quartet Books

Hysterectomy, Suzie Hayman. Sheldon Press

Hysterectomy and HRT, ed. John Studd & Linda Edwards. Martin Dunitz

Let's Get Things Moving – overcoming constipation, Pauline Chiarelli & Sue Markham. Neen Healthcare

Management of the Menopause, ed. Margaret Rees & David Purdie. BMS Publications, Marlow, Bucks

The Menopause and HRT, Kathy Abernethy. Saunders

Natural Menopause, Miriam Stoppard. Dorling Kindersley

Reinterpreting the Menopause, ed. Paul Komesaroff, Philippa Rothfield & Jeanne Daly. Routledge

Understanding Your Bowels, Kenneth Heaton. BMA Family Doctor Publications

Understanding Female Urinary Incontinence, Linda Cardozo, Philip Toozs-Hobson. BMA Family Doctor Publications

Understanding Hysterectomy and the Alternatives, Christine West. BMA Family Doctor Publications

Understanding Menopause and HRT, Anne MacGregor. BMA Family Doctor Publications

Women and Cancer, Giselle Moore & Lois Almadrones. Jones & Bartlett Publishers

Women's Waterworks: Curing Incontinence, Pauline Chiarelli. Neen Healthcare